WALL PILATES FOR BEGINNERS

A STEP-BY-STEP GUIDE TO BUILD STRENGTH AND BALANCE WITH CONFIDENCE

RICHARD E. MARSHALL

CONTENTS:

Wall Hamstring Stretch

Wall Chest Stretch

Wall Quad Stretch

Wall Shoulder Stretch

Wall Spinal Twist

Wall Hip Flexor Stretch

Wall Wrist Stretch

Wall Pigeon Stretch

Wall Standing Forward Fold

Wall Ankle Circles

Wall Standing Quadriceps Stretch

Wall Crossover Crunches

Wall Reverse Fly

Wall Single-Leg Balance

Wall Lateral Leg Lifts

Wall Single-Leg Deadlift

Wall Plank Knee Tucks

Wall Seated Spinal Twist

Wall Lunge Stretch

Wall Single-Leg Calf Raises

Wall Plank Hold

Wall Hamstring Press

Wall Reverse Lunges

INTRODUCTION

Welcome to the world of Wall Pilates, where you'll discover a unique and transformative approach to fitness. Picture this: You stand in front of the wall, ready to embark on a journey of self-discovery, strength, and alignment. As you gaze at the smooth surface, you can't help but feel a sense of anticipation for what lies ahead.

Imagine the wall as your supportive partner on this Pilates adventure, providing stability, feedback, and an opportunity to deepen your mind-body connection. With each exercise, you'll learn to rely on the wall's presence as a pillar of strength, guiding you through movements that will enhance your flexibility, tone your muscles, and promote overall well-being.

In this practice, you'll discover that Wall Pilates is more than just a workout. It's a holistic approach that integrates the principles of Pilates with the unique support of the wall. By aligning your body, engaging your core, and connecting with your breath, you'll unlock a new level of strength and stability.

As you delve into Wall Pilates, you'll find that it offers a wide range of benefits. It helps to improve posture, enhance muscular endurance, increase flexibility, and promote body awareness. Moreover, it is a low-impact exercise method, making it suitable for beginners or those recovering from injuries.

Throughout your journey, you'll learn to focus on quality of movement rather than quantity, emphasizing precision and control. The wall will become your anchor, allowing you to explore and deepen your understanding of each exercise, ensuring proper alignment and maximizing the effectiveness of your movements.

By practicing Wall Pilates consistently, you'll not only strengthen your body but also cultivate a deeper connection with yourself. You'll develop a heightened awareness of your body's capabilities, empowering you to move with grace and intention throughout your daily life.

So, as you take your first step towards Wall Pilates, remember to embrace this practice with an open mind and a willingness to challenge yourself. Each session offers an opportunity to grow stronger, more balanced, and aligned.

Get ready to embark on this journey of transformation. The wall awaits your presence, ready to guide you towards a more vibrant and harmonious you.

LET THE ADVENTURE BEGIN!

Prioritizing Your Well-being in Wall Pilates

When engaging in any physical activity, including Wall Pilates, it is crucial to prioritize your safety and well-being. By following these safety guidelines and taking necessary precautions, you can minimize the risk of injury and ensure a positive and fulfilling experience. Remember, your health and comfort should always be at the forefront of your practice.

Consult with a healthcare professional: Before starting any new exercise program, it's advisable to consult with a healthcare professional, especially if you have any pre-existing medical conditions, injuries, or concerns. They can provide personalized guidance based on your specific needs and ensure that Wall Pilates is suitable for you.

Choose a suitable space: Find a dedicated space for your Wall Pilates practice that is clear of any obstacles or hazards. Ensure that the wall is clean, stable, and securely mounted. Remove any sharp objects, slippery surfaces, or potential tripping hazards from the area.

Wear appropriate attire: Dress in comfortable, breathable clothing that allows for a full range of movement. Avoid wearing loose or baggy clothing that may interfere with your exercises or get caught on the wall or equipment.

Warm up and cool down: Always incorporate a warm-up and cool-down routine into your Wall Pilates practice. Start with gentle movements to increase blood flow and prepare your muscles for the exercises ahead. After your session, perform stretches to promote flexibility and aid in muscle recovery.

Start with beginner-friendly exercises: If you are new to Wall Pilates, begin with beginner-friendly exercises and gradually progress to more advanced movements as you gain strength, flexibility, and familiarity with the practice. This progressive approach allows your body to adapt and reduces the risk of strain or overexertion.

Listen to your body: Pay close attention to how your body feels during each exercise. Never push through sharp or intense pain. Discomfort, mild muscle soreness, and fatigue are normal, but if something feels wrong or causes significant pain, stop the exercise and seek guidance from a qualified instructor or healthcare professional.

Maintain proper form and alignment:
Focus on maintaining proper form and alignment throughout your Wall Pilates practice. Follow the instructions carefully, engage your core muscles, and be mindful of your posture. Proper alignment reduces the risk of strain on joints and ensures optimal muscle engagement.

Modify when necessary: Don't hesitate to modify exercises to suit your individual needs and abilities. Use props or modifications suggested by your instructor to adapt exercises to your current fitness level. Progress gradually, and only attempt advanced exercises when you feel ready and confident.

Stay hydrated: Hydration is important during any physical activity. Have a water bottle nearby and drink water before, during, and after your Wall Pilates session to stay adequately hydrated.

Breathe and relax: Maintain a relaxed and rhythmic breathing pattern throughout your practice. Avoid holding your breath, as proper breathing enhances the mind-body connection and helps release tension.

Seek professional guidance: If you're new to Wall Pilates or unsure about proper technique, consider seeking guidance from a certified Pilates instructor. They can provide personalized instruction, correct your form, and ensure that you're performing the exercises safely and effectively.

Remember, safety should always be a priority in your Wall Pilates practice. By following these guidelines, listening to your body, and seeking professional guidance when needed, you can enjoy the many benefits of Wall Pilates while minimizing the risk of injury. Prioritize your well-being, and let the wall be your trusted partner on your journey to strength, balance, and overall vitality.

WALL PILATES FOR BEGINNERS

Welcome to Wall Pilates for beginners! In this comprehensive guide, we will explore the procedure in a detailed bullet-point format, ensuring that you have a clear understanding of each exercise and its specific targets. Let's dive in and experience the transformative power of Wall Pilates together!

The primary objectives of Wall Pilates for beginners are:

Core Strengthening: By engaging your deep abdominal muscles, Wall Pilates helps to develop a strong and stable core, which is essential for supporting your spine and maintaining proper posture.

Alignment and Posture: Wall Pilates emphasizes proper alignment and encourages good posture, leading to improved body awareness and reduced strain on your joints.

Flexibility and Range of Motion: Regular Wall Pilates practice promotes flexibility, increases your range of motion, and enhances muscular balance, resulting in improved overall functional movement.

Procedure:

March in place to elevate your heart rate and warm up your muscles.

Perform shoulder rolls to release tension and prepare your upper body.

Engage in gentle spinal movements, such as forward and backward bends, to mobilize your spine.

Positioning and Alignment:

Procedure:

Stand with your back against the wall, feet hip-width apart, and a few inches away from the wall.

Ensure proper alignment of the head, shoulders, hips, and heels against the wall.

Breathing:

Procedure:

Establish a deep diaphragmatic breath pattern: inhale deeply through your nose and exhale fully through your mouth.

Maintain this rhythmic breathing throughout the exercises to enhance the mind-body connection.

Wall Squats (Targets: Lower Body Strength):

Procedure:

Slide down the wall into a squat position, aligning your knees with your ankles.

Hold the squat for a few seconds, engaging your quadriceps and gluteal muscles.

Push through your heels to stand back up, activating your hamstrings and core.

Repeat for 8-10 repetitions, focusing on proper alignment and controlled movements.

Wall Roll-Downs (Targets: Spinal Mobility and Hamstring Stretch):

Procedure:

Stand with your back against the wall and slowly roll down one vertebra at a time, keeping knees slightly bent.

Allow your hands to slide down the wall as you reach a comfortable stretch in your hamstrings.

Hold the stretch for a moment, engaging your core and focusing on breath.

Roll back up to a standing position, maintaining control and initiating the movement from your core.

Repeat 6-8 times, enjoying the sensation of spinal articulation and hamstring release.

Wall Angels (Targets: Upper Back Strength and Posture):

Procedure:

Stand against the wall with your arms bent at 90 degrees, elbows and wrists in contact with the wall.

Slide your arms up and down the wall, maintaining contact with elbows, wrists, and the back of your hands.

Focus on engaging your upper back muscles, promoting better posture and shoulder stability.

Perform 10-12 repetitions, emphasizing smooth and controlled movements.

Wall Plank (Targets: Core Strength and Stability):

Procedure:

Assume a plank position with your hands on the wall, shoulder-width apart.

Create a straight line from your head to your heels, engaging your core and gluteal muscles.

Hold this position for 20-30 seconds, gradually increasing duration as you gain strength.

Focus on maintaining proper alignment and breathing deeply throughout the exercise.

Cool-down and Stretching:

Procedure:

Engage in gentle movements to cool down your body, such as marching in place or light walking.

Perform stretches to elongate and relax your muscles, focusing on the hamstrings, quadriceps, chest, shoulders, and back.

Hold each stretch for 20-30 seconds, breathing deeply and allowing your body to unwind.

Wall Calf Raises (Targets: Calves and Ankle Stability):

Procedure:

Stand facing the wall with your hands resting lightly against it for support.

Rise up onto your toes, lifting your heels off the ground while maintaining a tall posture.

Controlled heel lowering is required as you stand back up.

Repeat for 10-12 repetitions, focusing on activating your calf muscles and improving ankle stability.

Wall Bridge (Targets: Glutes and Hamstrings):

Procedure:

Lie on your back with your feet against the wall and knees bent.

Press your feet into the wall as you lift your hips off the ground, forming a bridge position.

Squeeze your glutes and engage your hamstrings to maintain the bridge.

Slowly lower your hips back down to the ground, maintaining control throughout the movement.

Repeat for 8-10 repetitions, emphasizing the activation of your glutes and hamstrings.

Wall Side Leg Lifts (Targets: Hip Abductors):

Procedure:

Stand sideways to the wall with your hand lightly touching it for balance.

Lift your outside leg laterally, keeping your core engaged and maintaining proper alignment.

Lower the leg back down with control.

Repeat for 10-12 repetitions on each side, focusing on strengthening your hip abductor muscles.

Wall Push-Ups (Targets: Upper Body Strength):

Procedure:

Stand facing the wall with your arms extended and hands placed shoulder-width apart against the wall.

Bend your elbows, lowering your chest towards the wall while maintaining a straight body alignment.

Push back to the starting position, engaging your chest, shoulders, and triceps.

Repeat for 8-10 repetitions, adjusting the difficulty by adjusting your distance from the wall.

Wall Rotation (Targets: Core and Obliques):

Procedure:

Stand with your feet hip-width apart and your arms extended in front of you, pressed against the wall.

Rotate your torso to one side, pivoting from your waist while keeping your hips facing forward.

Return to the center and repeat the rotation to the other side.

Perform 8-10 repetitions on each side, focusing on engaging your core and oblique muscles.

Wall Leg Press (Targets: Quadriceps and Glutes):

Procedure:

Stand facing the wall with your hands resting lightly against it for support.

Lift one leg off the ground and press it straight back, engaging your quadriceps and glutes.

Return the foot to the ground with control and repeat the movement on the other leg.

Perform 10-12 repetitions on each leg, emphasizing the activation of your quadriceps and glutes.

Wall Abdominal Crunches (Targets: Abdominals):

Procedure:

Sit on the floor with your back against the wall, knees bent, and feet flat on the ground.

Engage your core as you lift your upper body off the ground, sliding your hands towards your knees.

Slowly lower your upper body back down to the ground, maintaining control throughout the movement.

Repeat for 10-12 repetitions, focusing on engaging your abdominal muscles and avoiding strain on your neck.

Wall Hamstring Curls (Targets: Hamstrings):

Procedure:

Lie on your back with your feet against the wall, knees bent, and arms relaxed by your sides.

Engage your hamstrings to slide your heels along the wall towards your glutes, lifting your hips off the ground.

Slowly extend your legs back out, returning to the starting position with control.

Repeat for 10-12 repetitions, emphasizing the activation of your hamstrings.

Wall Tricep Dips (Targets: Triceps):

Procedure:

Stand with your back against the wall and place your hands on the wall behind you at shoulder height.

Bend your elbows, lowering your body towards the wall while keeping your back close to it.

To extend your arms and get back to the beginning position, push through your hands.

Perform 8-10 repetitions, focusing on engaging your triceps throughout the movement.

Wall Side Plank (Targets: Core and Obliques):

Procedure:

Stand sideways to the wall and place your forearm against it, aligning your elbow with your shoulder.

Extend your legs out to the side, forming a straight line from head to heels.

Engage your core and lift your hips off the ground, creating a side plank position.

Hold for 20-30 seconds on each side, focusing on stability and alignment.

Wall Scapular Retraction (Targets: Upper Back and Posture):

Procedure:

Stand with your back against the wall and your arms extended in front of you.

Retract your shoulder blades toward your spine by squeezing them together.

Hold for a few seconds, feeling the engagement of your upper back muscles.

Relax and repeat for 8-10 repetitions, promoting improved upper back strength and posture.

Wall Lunges (Targets: Quadriceps and Glutes):

Procedure:

Stand facing away from the wall with your hands resting lightly against it for support.

Take a step forward with one foot and lower your body into a lunge position, ensuring your knee aligns with your ankle.

To get back to the beginning position, drive through your front heel.

Repeat for 8-10 repetitions on each leg, focusing on engaging your quadriceps and glutes.

Wall Shoulder Press (Targets: Shoulders and Upper Body Strength):

Procedure:

Stand facing the wall with your feet hip-width apart and your arms bent at 90 degrees, palms against the wall.

Press your hands into the wall, extending your arms overhead.

Slowly lower your hands back down to the starting position.

Repeat for 8-10 repetitions, emphasizing the activation of your shoulder muscles.

Wall Hamstring Stretch:

Procedure:

Lie on your back with your glutes against the wall and extend one leg up against the wall.

Keep your opposite leg extended on the floor or bend it for added comfort.

Hold the stretch for 20-30 seconds, feeling a gentle stretch in your hamstrings.

On the other side, repeat the stretch by switching legs.

Wall Chest Stretch:

Procedure:

Stand facing the wall with your arm extended to the side and lightly placed against it.

Gently rotate your body away from the wall, feeling a stretch in your chest and shoulder.

Hold the stretch for 20-30 seconds, focusing on deepening the stretch with each breath.

Repeat the stretch on the other side, maintaining balance and symmetry.

Wall Quad Stretch:

Procedure:

Stand facing the wall and use one hand to lightly touch it for support.

Bend one knee and bring your foot towards your glutes, reaching back with the same-side hand to grasp your ankle or foot.

Feel a stretch in your front thigh as you slowly pull your foot towards your glutes.

Hold the stretch for 20-30 seconds and repeat on the other leg, maintaining balance and stability.

Wall Shoulder Stretch:

Procedure:

Stand with your side against the wall and extend your arm straight out, palm against the wall.

Slowly rotate your body away from the wall, feeling a stretch in your shoulder and chest.

Hold the stretch for 20-30 seconds, focusing on maintaining proper alignment and breathing deeply.

Repeat the stretch on the other side, promoting balance and flexibility.

Wall Spinal Twist:

Procedure:

Stand with your back against the wall and your feet hip-width apart.

Place your hands on your hips and gently rotate your torso to one side, pivoting from your waist.

Keep your hips and feet facing forward, feeling a gentle twist in your spine.

Hold the stretch for 20-30 seconds, emphasizing breath and relaxation.

Repeat the stretch to the other side, promoting spinal mobility and release.

Wall Hip Flexor Stretch:

Procedure:

Kneel down facing away from the wall with one knee on the ground and the other foot against the wall, creating a lunge position.

Place your hands on your hips and gently lean forward, feeling a stretch in the front of your hip and thigh.

Hold the stretch for 20-30 seconds, focusing on maintaining balance and stability.

Switch legs and repeat the stretch on the other side, promoting balanced flexibility.

Wall Wrist Stretch:

Procedure:

Stand facing the wall with your arms extended, palms pressed against the wall at shoulder height.

Gently lean your body weight forward, keeping your palms against the wall and feeling a stretch in your wrists and forearms.

Hold the stretch for 20-30 seconds, focusing on relaxing the muscles and promoting wrist mobility.

Release the stretch slowly and repeat if needed, maintaining proper alignment and control.

Wall Pigeon Stretch:

Procedure:

Stand facing the wall and place both hands against it at shoulder height.

Take a step back and lift one leg, bending the knee and resting the outer ankle against the opposite thigh.

Gently lean into the wall, feeling a stretch in your hip and glutes.

Hold the stretch for 20-30 seconds, focusing on breath and relaxation.

Switch legs and repeat the stretch on the other side, promoting hip flexibility and release.

Wall Standing Forward Fold:

Procedure:

Stand facing the wall and place your hands against it at shoulder height.

Slowly hinge forward from your hips, allowing your torso to fold towards the ground.

Relax your neck and shoulders, feeling a gentle stretch in your hamstrings and back.

Hold the stretch for 20-30 seconds, focusing on breath and letting go of tension.

Slowly rise back up to a standing position, maintaining control and alignment.

Wall Ankle Circles:

Procedure:

Stand facing the wall and place your hands lightly against it for support.

Lift one foot off the ground and draw circles with your ankle, focusing on smooth and controlled movements.

Perform 10-12 circles in one direction, then switch directions.

Repeat the ankle circles on the other foot, promoting ankle mobility and flexibility.

Wall Standing Quadriceps Stretch:

Procedure:

Stand facing the wall and place one hand against it for balance.

Bend one knee and reach back with the same-side hand to grasp your ankle or foot.

Gently pull your foot towards your glutes, feeling a stretch in the front of your thigh.

Hold the stretch for 20-30 seconds, focusing on breath and maintaining stability.

Switch legs and repeat the stretch on the other side, promoting balance and flexibility.

Wall Crossover Crunches (Targets: Obliques and Abdominals):

Procedure:

Lie on your back with your legs extended against the wall, forming a 90-degree angle with your body.

Place your hands behind your head and lift your upper body, twisting diagonally to bring your opposite elbow towards your knee.

Engage your obliques and abdominals as you perform the crunch.

Repeat for 10-12 repetitions on each side, alternating the twisting motion.

Wall Reverse Fly (Targets: Upper Back and Shoulders):

Procedure:

Stand facing the wall with your feet hip-width apart and your arms extended in front of you, hands lightly pressed against the wall.

Squeeze your shoulder blades together as you open your arms out to the sides, keeping them at shoulder height.

Engage your upper back muscles to perform the movement.

Return to the starting position with control.

Repeat for 8-10 repetitions, emphasizing the activation of your upper back and shoulders.

Wall Single-Leg Balance (Targets: Balance and Stability):

Procedure:

Stand facing the wall with your feet hip-width apart and your hands resting lightly against it for support.

Lift one leg off the ground and find your balance, maintaining a tall posture.

Hold the position for 20-30 seconds, engaging your core and focusing on stability.

Switch legs and repeat the balance exercise on the other side.

Wall Lateral Leg Lifts (Targets: Hip Abductors and Glutes):

Procedure:

Stand facing the wall with your hands lightly resting against it for balance.

Lift one leg out to the side, keeping it straight and engaging your hip abductors.

Lower the leg back down with control.

Repeat for 10-12 repetitions on each leg, focusing on strengthening your hip abductor muscles.

Wall Single-Leg Deadlift (Targets: Hamstrings and Glutes):

Procedure:

Stand facing the wall with your feet hip-width apart and your hands lightly resting against it for support.

Shift your weight onto one leg and hinge forward at the hips, extending your opposite leg straight back.

Maintain a slight bend in the standing leg and keep your back straight as you reach a comfortable stretch in your hamstrings.

Engage your glutes and hamstrings to return to the starting position.

Repeat for 8-10 repetitions on each leg, focusing on balance and controlled movements.

Wall Plank Knee Tucks (Targets: Core and Hip Flexors):

Procedure:

Assume a plank position with your hands on the floor and your feet against the wall, forming an inclined angle.

Engage your core and bring one knee towards your chest, using your hip flexors to tuck it in.

Extend the leg back to the starting position and repeat the movement on the other leg.

Perform 8-10 knee tucks on each side, focusing on maintaining stability and control.

Wall Seated Spinal Twist (Targets: Spinal Mobility and Stretch):

Your legs should be out in front of you while you sit on the floor with your back against the wall.

Bend one knee and place the foot on the outside of the opposite leg.

Twist your torso towards the bent knee, using the wall for support and feeling a gentle stretch in your spine.

Hold the stretch for 20-30 seconds, focusing on breath and relaxation.

Repeat the twist on the other side, promoting spinal mobility and release.

Wall Lunge Stretch (Targets: Hip Flexors and Quadriceps):

Procedure:

Stand facing away from the wall and take a step back with one foot, bending the knee to lower into a lunge position.

Place your hands on the wall for support and lean your body weight forward, feeling a stretch in the front of your hip and thigh.

Hold the stretch for 20-30 seconds and switch legs, maintaining balance and stability.

Repeat the lunge stretch on the other side, promoting flexibility in the hip flexors and quadriceps.

Wall Single-Leg Calf Raises (Targets: Calves and Ankle Stability):

Procedure:

Stand facing the wall with your hands resting lightly against it for support.

Lift one foot off the ground and rise up onto your toes on the standing leg, activating your calf muscles.

Lower your heel back down in a controlled manner.

Repeat for 10-12 repetitions on each leg, focusing on strengthening your calf muscles and improving ankle stability.

Wall Plank Hold (Targets: Core and Upper Body Strength):

Procedure:

Assume a plank position with your forearms against the wall and your feet extended behind you, forming a straight line from head to heels.

Engage your core, glutes, and shoulder muscles to hold the position.

Aim to hold the plank for 30-60 seconds, focusing on maintaining proper alignment and breath control.

As your strength increases, gradually lengthen the exercise.

Wall Hamstring Press (Targets: Hamstrings and Glutes):

Procedure:

Lie on your back with your feet against the wall, knees bent, and arms relaxed by your sides.

Engage your hamstrings and glutes to press your feet into the wall, lifting your hips off the ground.

Keep your core activated and maintain a straight line from your knees to your shoulders.

Slowly lower your hips back down to the ground with control.

Repeat for 8-10 repetitions, emphasizing the activation of your hamstrings and glutes.

Wall Reverse Lunges (Targets: Quadriceps, Glutes, and Balance):

Procedure:

Stand facing the wall with your hands lightly resting against it for support.

Take a step back with one foot, bending both knees to lower into a lunge position.

To get back to the starting position, press through the front heel.

Repeat for 8-10 repetitions on each leg, focusing on engaging your quadriceps, glutes, and maintaining balance.

Wall Plank Shoulder Taps (Targets: Core and Shoulder Stability):

Procedure:

Assume a plank position with your hands against the wall and your feet extended behind you, forming a straight line from head to heels.

Lift one hand off the wall and tap the opposite shoulder while maintaining a stable core and avoiding hip rotation.

Return the hand to the wall and repeat the movement on the other side.

Perform 10-12 shoulder taps on each side, focusing on stability and control.

Wall Side Bend (Targets: Obliques and Core):

Procedure:

Stand with your side against the wall and place your hand lightly on it for support.

Extend the arm above your head and gently lean towards the wall, feeling a stretch along the side of your body.

Engage your oblique muscles to return to the upright position.

Perform 8-10 repetitions on each side, emphasizing the activation of your obliques and maintaining proper alignment.

Wall Squats (Targets: Quadriceps, Glutes, and Lower Body Strength):

Procedure:

Your feet should be shoulder-width apart as you stand with your back to the wall.

Slide your body down the wall, bending your knees and lowering into a squat position.

Keep your knees aligned with your ankles and your back against the wall.

Hold the squat for 20-30 seconds, focusing on engaging your quadriceps and glutes.

Slowly rise back up to the starting position, maintaining control and proper form.

Wall Calf Stretches:

Procedure:

Stand facing the wall and place both hands against it at shoulder height.

Take a step back with one foot, keeping the heel on the ground and the knee straight.

Lean forward, feeling a stretch in your calf muscle.

Hold the stretch for 20-30 seconds and repeat on the other leg, focusing on breath and relaxation.

Wall Bridge (Targets: Glutes and Core):

Procedure:

Lie on your back with your feet against the wall, knees bent, and arms relaxed by your sides.

Engage your glutes and core to lift your hips off the ground, forming a bridge position.

Hold the bridge for 20-30 seconds, focusing on maintaining a straight line from your knees to your shoulders.

Lower your hips back down with control.

Repeat for 8-10 repetitions, emphasizing the activation of your glutes and core muscles.

Wall Bicep Curls (Targets: Biceps):

Procedure:

Stand facing the wall with your feet hip-width apart and your arms extended in front of you, palms pressed against the wall.

Bend your elbows, pulling your body towards the wall while keeping your back straight.

Engage your biceps to perform the curling movement.

Return to the starting position with control.

Repeat for 8-10 repetitions, focusing on the activation of your biceps.

CONCLUSION

Embracing the Benefits of Wall Pilates

Congratulations on completing your journey through the world of Wall Pilates! You have delved into a practice that goes beyond physical fitness, providing a pathway to strength, alignment, and holistic well-being. Through the support of the wall, you have discovered the power of precision, control, and mindful movement.

By engaging in Wall Pilates, you have experienced numerous benefits. Your posture has improved, allowing you to stand taller and move with grace and confidence. Your muscles have grown stronger, enhancing your stability and endurance. Flexibility has increased, granting you a greater range of motion and freedom in your body. And perhaps most importantly, you have cultivated a deeper connection between your mind and body, nurturing self-awareness and inner balance.

As you continue on your journey, remember to embrace the principles of Wall Pilates in all aspects of your life. Carry the lessons of alignment, breath control, and mindful movement beyond the wall, integrating them into

your daily routines and activities. Let the strength
and grace you have developed in your practice
become a part of who you are.